2021 Plant Based Cooking Guide

The New Plant Based Diet

Recipes Collection

Joanna Vinson

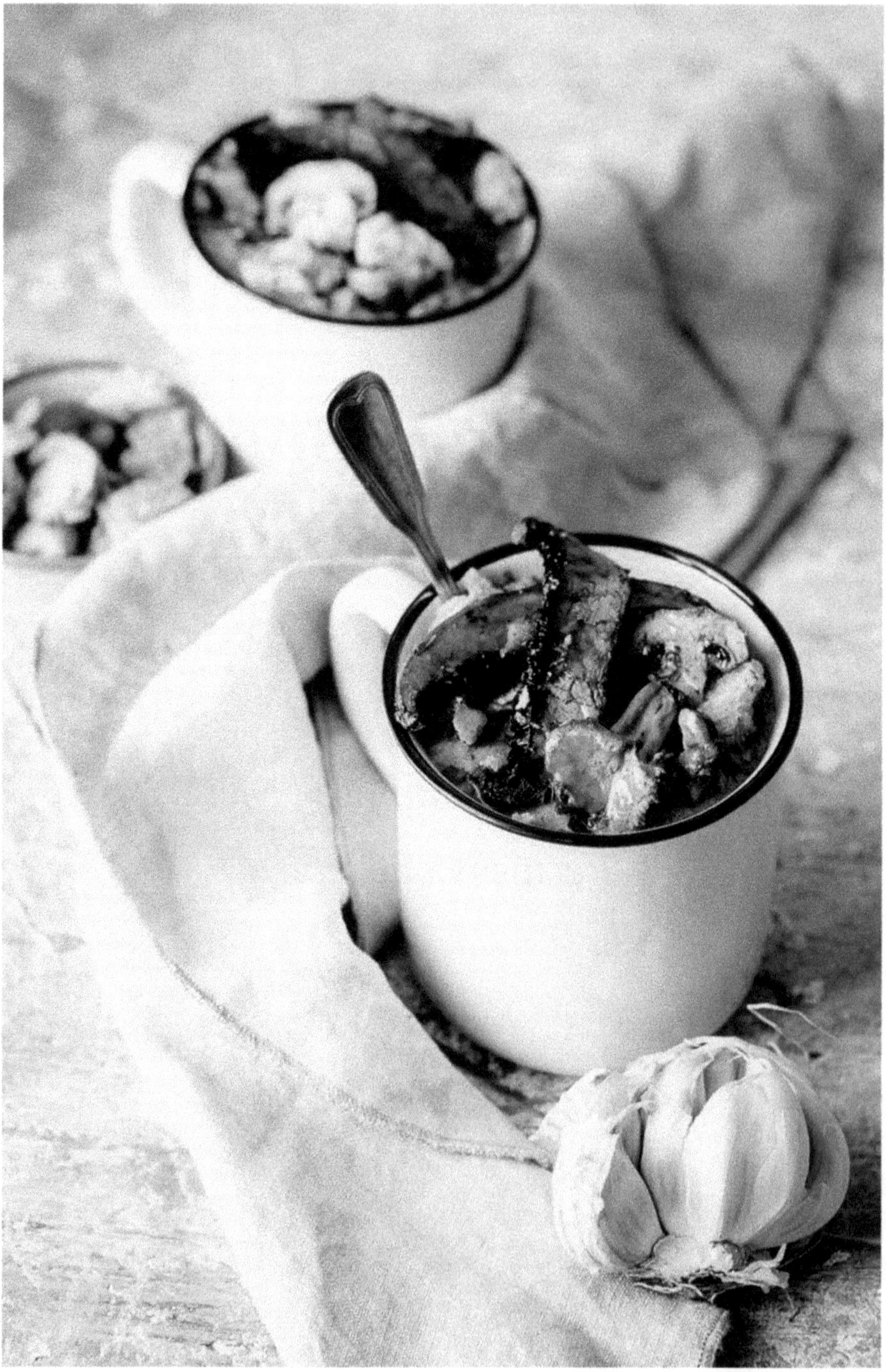

Table of Contents

Parsnip Ginger Soup with Tofu and Kale

Preparation Time: 10 minutes | Cooking Time: 20 minutes | Servings: 2

Ingredients:

- ½ tablespoon butter

- 1 small onion, diced

- 1 teaspoon ginger powder

- 1 teaspoon garlic powder

- ½ pound parsnip, cut into small coins

- ½ teaspoon cumin

- ½ teaspoon ground coriander

- ¼ teaspoon ground turmeric

- 1 1/2 cups of vegetable broth

- ½ cup of soy milk

- ½ teaspoon honey

- ½ fresh lime

- 1 cup tofu, diced into cubes

- 1 handful of fresh kale

Directions:

- Set the Pressure pot to Sauté and add butter, add tofu and cook it for 5 minutes. Keep aside.

- After adding onions. Cook for 5-10 minutes until the onion begins to soften.

- Add the garlic and ginger powder to the pot and stir until fragrant.

- Combine the parsnip, cumin, coriander powder, and turmeric powder in the Pressure pot. Stir

well.

- Pour in the broth and lock the lid. Turn the vent to seal, press Cancel, and manually cook on High Pressure for 5 minutes.

- After the 5 minutes, do a manual release.

- Add the soy milk and honey if using to the Pressure pot. Allow the mixture to cool slightly and then use an immersion blender or other mixer to puree until smooth. Season with salt, pepper, and a squeeze of lime.

• Stir the fresh kale into the still slightly warm soup. The kale should wilt on its own, but you can also warm it up together for the right temperature. Add the tof and enjoy!

Nutrition:

Calories 303 | Total Fat 10. 5g | Saturated Fat 3. 3g | Cholesterol 8mg | Sodium 478mg | Total Carbohydrate 38. 9g | Dietary Fiber 9. 2g | Total Sugars 12. 6g | Protein 18. 1g

Mushroom Soup

Preparation Time: 10 minutes | Cooking Time: 25 minutes | Servings: 2

Ingredients:

- 1 teaspoon avocado oil

- ½ medium onion, chopped

- ½ large leek stalk, chopped

- ½ large zucchini peeled & chopped

- 1 teaspoon garlic powder

- 8 ounces of mushrooms sliced

- ½ teaspoon dried rosemary

- ¼ teaspoon ground pepper

- 1 1/2 cups vegetable broth

- ¼ teaspoon salt

- ½ cup almond milk

Directions:

• Set the Pressure pot to Sauté mode. Heat the avocado oil, then add the onion, leek, and zucchini. Sauté the vegetables, stirring occasionally, until starting to soften, 3 to 4 minutes.

• Add the garlic powder, mushrooms, rosemary, and pepper. Cook until the mushrooms are starting to release their liquid, 2 to 3 minutes. Stir in the broth and salt.

• Put the lid on the Pressure pot, close the steam vent, and set it to High Pressure using the Manual setting. Decrease the time to 10 minutes. It will take the Pressure pot about 10 minutes to reach pressure.

• Once the time is up, carefully release the steam using the Quick-release valve.

• Transfer half of the soup to the blender, add the almond milk, hold on the top and blend until almost smooth, stopping the blender and opening the lid occasionally to release the steam. Transfer the pureed soup to a pot or bowl.

Nutrition:

Calories228 | Total Fat 15. 9g | Saturated Fat 13g | Cholesterol 0mg | Sodium 702mg | Total Carbohydrate 17. 5g | Dietary Fiber 4. 8g | Total Sugars 8. 1g | Protein 9. 3g

Seitan Stew with Barley

Preparation Time: 10 minutes | Cooking Time: 20 minutes | Servings: 2

Ingredients:

- 1 teaspoon coconut oil

- ½ onion chopped

- 1 parsnip cut into thin half-circles

- 1 leek stalks diced

- 1 teaspoon garlic minced

- 1 teaspoon dried basil

- ½ teaspoons dried parsley

- 1 1/2 tablespoons tomato paste

- 2 cups vegetable broth

- 1 cup seitan

- 1 cup dry barley

- ½ teaspoon salt

- ½ teaspoon ground pepper

Directions:

• Set the Pressure pot to Sauté mode. Heat the coconut oil, then add the onion, parsnips, and leek. Sauté the vegetables, stirring occasionally, until starting to soften, 3 to 4 minutes.

• Add the garlic, basil, parsley, and tomato paste. Cook, stirring constantly, for 1 minute.

• Pour in the vegetable broth and stir to combine.

• Add the seitan, barley, and salt and pepper to the Pressure pot.

• Put the lid on the Pressure pot, close the steam vent, and set it to High Pressure using the Manual setting. Set the time to 20 minutes.

• Once the time is expired, use Natural-release for 10 minutes, then quickly release.

• Serve soup with salt and pepper to taste.

Nutrition:

Calories 376 | Total Fat 5. 8g | Saturated Fat 2. 9g | Cholesterol 0mg | Sodium 1600mg | Total Carbohydrate 57. 9g | Dietary Fiber 13. 7g | Total Sugars 8. 2g | Protein 23. 5g

Cottage Cheese Soup

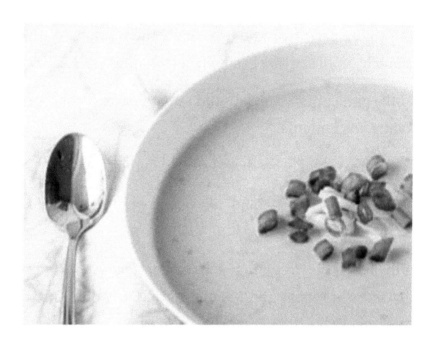

Preparation Time: 10 minutes | Cooking Time: 35 minutes | Servings: 2

Ingredients:

- 1 stalks leek, diced

- 1 tablespoon bell pepper, diced

- ¼ cup Swiss chard, sliced into strips

- 1/8 cup fresh kale

- 1 eggplant

- ½ tablespoon avocado oil

- 1/8 cup button mushrooms, diced

- 1 small onion, diced

- ½ cup cottage cheese

- 2 cups vegetable broth

- 1 bay leaf

- ½ teaspoon salt

- ¼ teaspoon garlic, minced

- 1/8 teaspoon paprika

Directions:

• Place leek, bell pepper, Swiss chard, eggplant, and kale into a medium bowl, set aside in a separate medium bowl.

• Press the Sauté button and add the avocado oil to Pressure pot. Once the oil is hot, add mushrooms and onion. Sauté for 4–6 minutes until the onion is translucent and fragrant.

• Add leek, bell pepper, Swiss chard, and kale to Pressure pot. Cook for an additional 4 minutes. Press the Cancel button.

• Add diced cottage cheese, broth, bay leaf, and seasonings to Pressure pot. Click the lid closed. Press the Soup button and set the time for 20 minutes.

• When the timer beeps, allow a 10-minute natural release and quickly release the remaining pressure. Add eggplant on Keep Warm mode and cook for additional 10 minutes or until tender. Serve warm.

Nutrition:

Calories 212 | Total Fat 3. 6g | Saturated Fat 1. 2g | Cholesterol 5mg | Sodium 1603mg | Total Carbohydrate 30. 7g | Dietary Fiber 11. 9g | Total Sugars 12. 7g | Protein 17g

Fresh Corn & Red Pepper Stew

Preparation Time: 15 minutes | Cooking Time: 30 minutes | Servings: 2

Ingredients:

- 1 teaspoon coconut oil

- ¼ cup sweet onion, chopped,

- 1 1/2 cups fresh corn kernels

- 1 teaspoon garlic, minced

- 2 cups vegetable broth,

- ¼ teaspoon salt

- 1/8 cup coconut cream

- ½ tablespoon cornmeal

- ½ small red bell pepper, diced

- Enough water

Directions:

• Select the Sauté setting on the Pressure pot and heat the coconut oil. Add the onion, garlic, and salt and sauté for about 5 minutes, until the onion has softened and is translucent.

• Add the fresh corn, broth, water, bell pepper, and stir well.

• Lock lid and set the Pressure Release to Sealing. Press the Cancel button to reset the cooking program, then select the Soup/Broth setting and set the cooking time for 15 minutes at High Pressure.

• Meanwhile add water, coconut cream, and cornmeal.

• Let the pressure release naturally for at least 10 minutes, then move the Steam Release to Vent to release any remaining steam.

• Open the pot and stir in the cornmeal mixer into soup, then taste and adjust the seasoning with salt if needed.

Nutrition:

Calories 183 | Total Fat 8. 3g | Saturated Fat 5. 7g | Cholesterol 0mg | Sodium 1070mg | Total Carbohydrate 21. 8g | Dietary Fiber 3. 3g | Total Sugars 5. 8g | Protein 8. 4g

Zucchini & White Bean Stew

Preparation Time: 10 minutes | Cooking Time: 35 minutes | Servings: 2

Ingredients:

- ¼ ounce mushrooms

- 1 cup hot water

- ½ large zucchini

- 1 tablespoon coconut oil, divided

- 1 small onion, thinly sliced

- ½ teaspoon garlic powder

- ¼ teaspoons dried basil, crumbled

- 1 small (1-inch) cinnamon stick

- ¼ teaspoon salt

- 1/8 teaspoon freshly ground pepper

- 1 bay leaf

- 2 cups vegetable broth

- ¼ cup dried white beans, rinsed and soaked overnight and drained

- 1 tomato

- ¼ cup finely chopped fresh cilantro

Directions:

- Select the Sauté setting on the Pressure pot and heat ¼ tablespoon coconut oil. Add zucchini and roast it and keep aside.

- Add remaining coconut oil, add onion and sauté for about 5 minutes, until the onion has softened and is translucent. Add garlic powder, basil, cinnamon stick, salt, pepper, bay leaf, and the chopped mushrooms cook, stirring, for 1 minute add vegetable broth and add white beans and roast zucchini.

- Lock lid and set the Pressure Release to Sealing. Press the Cancel button to reset the cooking program, then select the Soup/Broth setting and set the cooking time for 25 minutes at High Pressure.

- Let the pressure release naturally for at least 10 minutes, then move the Steam Release to Vent to release any remaining steam.

- Open the pot and remove the cinnamon stick and bay leaf. Stir in tomatoes and cilantro.

Nutrition:

Calories 210 | Total Fat 7. 5g | Saturated Fat 6g | Cholesterol 0mg | Sodium 307mg | Total Carbohydrate 30. 9g | Dietary Fiber 11. 1g | Total Sugars 8g | Protein 8. 5g

Potato Tofu Soup

Preparation Time: 10 minutes | Cooking Time: 35 minutes | Servings: 2

Ingredients:

- ½ tablespoon olive oil

- ½ celery cleaned and sliced

- ½ teaspoon garlic powder

- 1 sweet potato peeled and cut into 2-inch cubes

- ½ large potato peeled and cut into 2-inch cubes

- ½ cup tofu

- 2 cups vegetable broth

- Juice from one lemon

- A handful of chopped parsley

- Salt and pepper

Directions:

• Hit the Sauté button and when it's hot, heat the olive oil in your Pressure pot and sauté the celery and garlic powder until they soften down, stirring often.

• Add in the potatoes, sweet potatoes, tofu, broth, salt, and pepper, and stir well.

• Lock lid, make sure the vent is sealed, and program for 6 minutes on High Pressure. You can do a Quick-release if you like or leave it to release on its own with soup like this it doesn't matter.

• Once the pressure is released, open the lid and throw in the parsley and add the lemon juice.

Nutrition:

Calories 216 | Total Fat 7. 6g | Saturated Fat 1. 5g | Cholesterol 0mg | Sodium 809mg | Total Carbohydrate 27. 2g | Dietary Fiber 3. 6g | Total Sugars 5. 2g | Protein 12. 2g

Tomato Gazpacho

Preparation Time: 2 Hours 25 minutes | Cooking Time: 15-60 minutes | Servings: 6

Ingredients:

• 2 Tablespoons + 1 Teaspoon Red Wine Vinegar, Divided

• ½ Teaspoon Pepper

• 1 Teaspoon Sea Salt

• 1 Avocado,

• ¼ Cup Basil, Fresh & Chopped

• 3 Tablespoons + 2 Teaspoons Olive Oil, Divided

• 1 Clove Garlic, crushed

• 1 Red Bell Pepper, Sliced & Seeded

• 1 Cucumber, Chunked

• 2 ½ lbs. Large Tomatoes, Cored & Chopped

Directions:

• Place half of your cucumber, bell pepper, and ¼ cup of each tomato in a bowl, covering. Set it in the fridge.

• Puree your remaining tomatoes, cucumber, and bell pepper with garlic, three tablespoons oil, two tablespoons of vinegar, sea salt, and black pepper into a blender, blending until smooth. Transfer it to a bowl, and chill for two hours.

• Chop the avocado, adding it to your chopped vegetables, adding your remaining oil, vinegar, salt, pepper, and basil.

• Ladle your tomato puree mixture into bowls, and serve with chopped vegetables as a salad.

Interesting Facts: Avocados themselves are ranked within the top five of the healthiest foods on the planet, so you know that the oil that is produced from them is too. It is loaded with healthy fats and essential fatty acids. Like race bran oil it is perfect to cook with as well! Bonus: Helps in the prevention of diabetes and lowers cholesterol levels.

Nutrition:

Calories 70 |Fat 2.7 g | Carbohydrates 13.8 g | Sugar 6.3 g | Protein 1.9 g | Cholesterol 0 mg

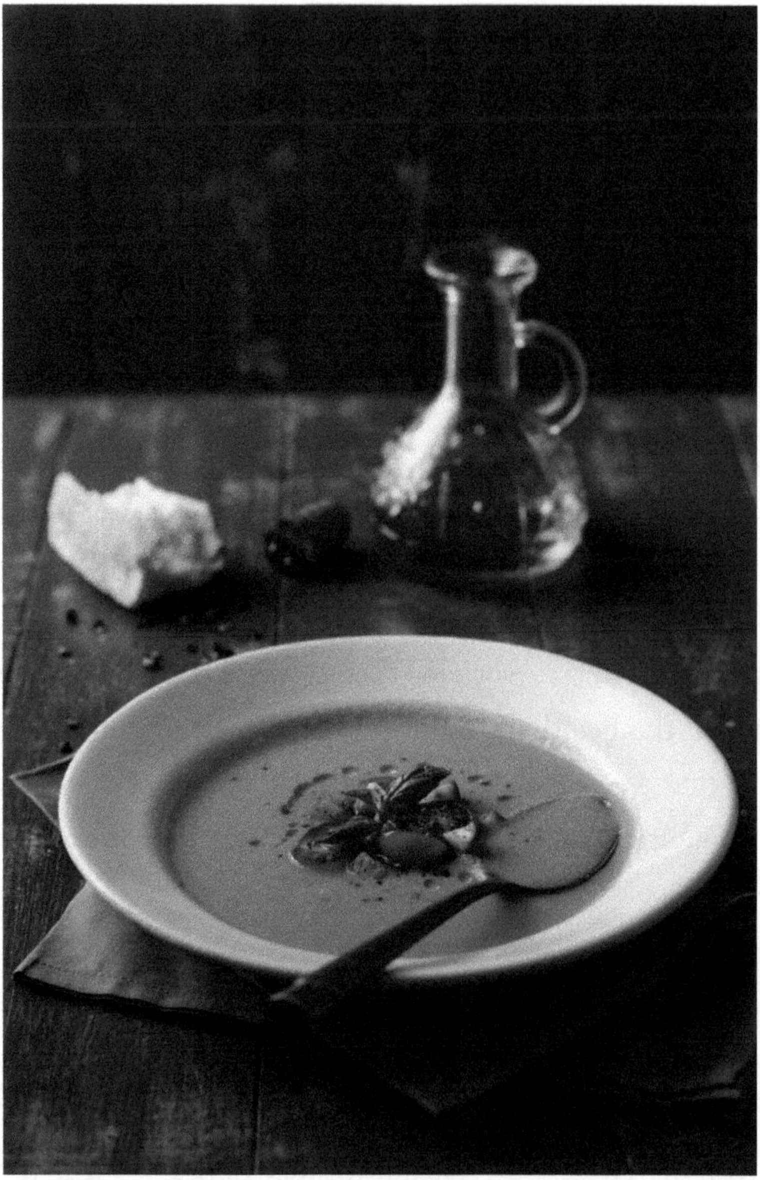

Tomato Pumpkin Soup

Preparation Time: 25 minutes | Cooking Time: 15-60 minutes | Servings: 4

Ingredients:

- 2 cups pumpkin, diced

- 1/2 cup tomato, chopped

- 1/2 cup onion, chopped

- 1 1/2 tsp curry powder

- 1/2 tsp paprika

- 2 cups vegetable stock

- 1 tsp olive oil

- 1/2 tsp garlic, minced

Directions:

- In a saucepan, add oil, garlic, and onion and sauté for 3 minutes over medium heat.

- Add remaining ingredients into the saucepan and bring to boil.

- Reduce heat and cover and simmer for 10 minutes.

- Puree the soup using a blender until smooth.

- Stir well and serve warm.

Nutrition:

Calories 70 |Fat 2.7 g |Carbohydrates 13.8 g |Sugar 6.3 g |Protein 1.9 g |Cholesterol 0 mg

Cauliflower Spinach Soup

Preparation Time: 45 minutes | Cooking Time: 15-60 minutes | Servings: 5

Ingredients:

- 1/2 cup unsweetened coconut milk

- 5 oz fresh spinach, chopped

- 5 watercress, chopped

- 8 cups vegetable stock

- 1 lb cauliflower, chopped

- Salt

Directions:

• Add stock and cauliflower in a large saucepan and bring to boil over medium heat for 15 minutes.

• Add spinach and watercress and cook for another 10 minutes.

• Remove from heat and puree the soup using a blender until smooth.

• Add coconut milk and stir well. Season with salt.

• Stir well and serve hot.

Nutrition:

Calories 153 | Fat 8.3 g | Carbohydrates 8.7 g | Sugar 4.3 g |Protein 11.9 g | Cholesterol 0 mg

Avocado Mint Soup

Preparation Time: 10 minutes | Cooking Time: 15-60 minutes | Servings: 2

Ingredients:

- 1 medium avocado, peeled, pitted, and cut into pieces

- 1 cup of coconut milk

- 2 romaine lettuce leaves

- 20 fresh mint leaves

- 1 tbsp fresh lime juice

- 1/8 tsp salt

Directions:

- Add all ingredients into the blender and blend until smooth. The soup should be thick not as a puree.

- Pour into the serving bowls and place in the refrigerator for 10 minutes.

- Stir well and serve chilled.

Nutrition:

Calories 268 | Fat 25.6 g | Carbohydrates 10.2 g | Sugar 0.6 g | Protein 2.7 g | Cholesterol 0 mg

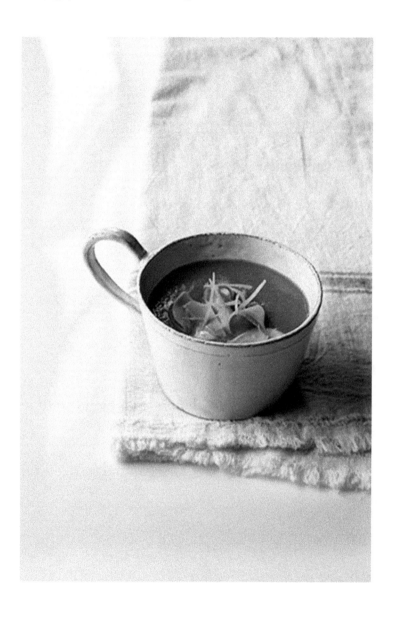

Creamy Squash Soup

Preparation Time: 35 minutes | Cooking Time: 15-60 minutes | Servings: 8

Ingredients:

• 3 cups butternut squash, chopped

• 1 ½ cups unsweetened coconut milk

• 1 tbsp coconut oil

• 1 tsp dried onion flakes

• 1 tbsp curry powder

• 4 cups of water

• 1 garlic clove

• 1 tsp kosher salt

Directions:

• Add squash, coconut oil, onion flakes, curry powder, water, garlic, and salt into a large saucepan. Bring to boil over high heat.

• Turn heat to medium and simmer for 20 minutes.

• Puree the soup using a blender until smooth. Return soup to the saucepan and stir in coconut milk and cook for 2 minutes.

• Stir well and serve hot.

Nutrition:

Calories 146 | Fat 12.6 g | Carbohydrates 9.4 g | Sugar 2.8 g | Protein 1.7 g | Cholesterol 0 mg

Zucchini Soup

Preparation Time: 20 minutes | Cooking Time: 15-60 minutes | Servings: 8

Ingredients:

• 2 ½ lbs zucchini, peeled and sliced

• 1/3 cup basil leaves

• 4 cups vegetable stock

• 4 garlic cloves, chopped

• 2 tbsp olive oil

• 1 medium onion, diced

• Pepper

• Salt

Directions:

• Heat olive oil in a pan over medium-low heat.

• Add zucchini and onion and sauté until softened. Add garlic and sauté for a minute.

• Add vegetable stock and simmer for 15 minutes.

• Remove from heat. Stir in basil and puree the soup using a blender until smooth and creamy. Season with pepper and salt.

• Stir well and serve.

Nutrition:

Calories 62 | Fat 4 g | Carbohydrates 6.8 g | Sugar 3.3 g | Protein 2 g | Cholesterol 0 mg

Creamy Celery Soup

Preparation Time: 40 minutes | Cooking Time: 15-60 minutes | Servings: 4

Ingredients:

- 6 cups celery
- ½ tsp dill
- 2 cups of water
- 1 cup of coconut milk
- 1 onion, chopped
- Pinch of salt

Directions:

- Add all ingredients into the electric pot and stir well.
- Cover the electric pot with the lid and select the soup setting.
- Release pressure using a quick-release method than opening the lid.
- Puree the soup using an immersion blender until smooth and creamy.

• Stir well and serve warm.

Nutrition:

Calories 174 | Fat 14.6 g | Carbohydrates 10.5 g | Sugar 5.2 g | Protein 2.8 g | Cholesterol 0 mg

Avocado Cucumber Soup

Preparation Time: 40 minutes | Cooking Time: 15-60 minutes | Servings: 3

Ingredients:

• 1 large cucumber, peeled and sliced

• ¾ cup of water

• ¼ cup lemon juice

• 2 garlic cloves

• 6 green onion

• 2 avocados, pitted

• ½ tsp black pepper

• ½ tsp pink salt

Directions:

• Add all ingredients into the blender and blend until smooth and creamy.

• Place in the refrigerator for 30 minutes.

• Stir well and serve chilled.

Nutrition:

Calories 73 | Fat 3.7 g | Carbohydrates 9.2 g | Sugar 2.8 g | Protein 2.2 g | Cholesterol 0 mg

Quick Jackfruit and Bean Stew

Preparation Time: 10 minutes | Cooking Time: 10 minutes | Servings: 2

Ingredients:

- ½ cup jackfruit cut into 1-inch pieces

- ½ cup kidney bean rinsed and drained

- ½ cup pinto beans rinsed and drained

- 1 tomato

- ½ onion chopped

- 2 cup vegetable broth or water

- ½ orange juiced

- ½ teaspoon salt and pepper

- ½ teaspoon cumin

- 1 bay leaf

- Fresh basil

Directions:

• Combine kidney beans, jackfruit, pinto beans, tomato, onion, broth, orange juice, pepper, salt, cumin, and bay leaf in Pressure pot; mix them well.

• Lock lid in place and turn the valve to Sealing. Press Manual or Pressure Cooker; cook at High Pressure 6 minutes.

• When cooking is complete, use Natural-release for 5 minutes, then release remaining pressure.

• Press Sauté, cook for 3 to 5 minutes or until the stew thickens slightly, stirring frequently. Remove and discard bay leaf. Garnish with basil.

Nutrition:

Calories 222 | Total Fat 2. 3g | Saturated Fat 0. 6g | Cholesterol 0mg | Sodium 1617mg | Total Carbohydrate 38. 5g | Dietary Fiber 9. 2g | Total Sugars 5. 9g | Protein 13. 6g

Split Pea Soup

Preparation Time: 15 minutes | Cooking Time: 15 minutes | Servings: 2

Ingredients:

- ½ onion chopped

- 1 zucchini chopped

- ¼ stalk leek chopped

- 1 teaspoon garlic powder

- ¼ teaspoon dried basil

- 2 cups vegetable broth

- 1 cup of water

- 1 cup dried split peas rinsed and sorted

- ½ teaspoon salt

- ½ teaspoon black pepper

- 1 bay leaf

Directions:

• Press Sauté, add onion, zucchini, and leek to Pressure pot; cook and stir 5 minutes or until vegetables are softened. Add garlic powder and basil; cook and stir for 1 minute. Stir in broth and water. Add split peas, salt, pepper, and bay leaf; mix well.

• Lock lid and move pressure release valve to the Sealing position. Press Manual or Pressure

Cooker; cook at High Pressure 8 minutes.

• When cooking is complete, use Natural-release for 10 minutes, then release remaining

 pressure. Stir soup; remove and discard bay leaf.

Nutrition:

Calories118 | Total Fat 1. 7g | Saturated Fat 0. 4g | Cholesterol 0mg | Sodium 1358mg | Total Carbohydrate 16. 7g | Dietary Fiber 2. 3g | Total Sugars 3. 7g | Protein 9. 5g

Pasta Tofu Soup

Preparation Time: 10 minutes | Cooking Time: 10 minutes | Servings: 2

Ingredients:

- ½ tablespoon butter

- ½ teaspoon garlic ginger, crushed

- ¼ onion chopped

- ½ green chilies, finely chopped (or adjust to taste

- ½ big tomato, chopped

- Salt to taste

- ¼ cup pasta

- ½ cup of tofu cubes

- 2 cups water or broth as needed

- Cilantro to garnish

Directions:

• Put Pressure pot on Sauté mode High and add butter. Once butter is hot, add garlic ginger and fry until aromatic.

• Add onions and green chili, fry till edges of onions brown, then add tomatoes and fry for 2 to 3 minutes.

• Add the pasta and tofu. Mix gently.

• Add salt, and the water about 1/2 inch to 1 inch covering the pasta and mix well. Turn off the Sauté mode. Lock lid in place and turn the valve to Sealing.

• Do Manual (Pressure Cooker) High 5 to 6 minutes. Let it naturally release or quick release after 10 minutes in Warm mode.

• Garnish with cilantro if desired and serve hot.

Nutrition:

Calories 196 | Total Fat 9. 2g | Saturated Fat 2. 7g | Cholesterol 19mg | Sodium 161mg | Total Carbohydrate 18g | Dietary Fiber 4g | Total Sugars 3. 3g | Protein 13. 3g

Creamy Garlic Onion Soup

Preparation Time: 45 minutes | Cooking Time: 15-60 minutes | Servings: 4

Ingredients:

- 1 onion, sliced

- 4 cups vegetable stock

- 1 1/2 tbsp olive oil

- 1 shallot, sliced

- 2 garlic clove, chopped

- 1 leek, sliced

- Salt

Directions:

- Add stock and olive oil in a saucepan and bring to boil.

- Add remaining ingredients and stir well.

- Cover and simmer for 25 minutes.

- Puree the soup using an immersion blender until smooth.

• Stir well and serve warm.

Nutrition:

Calories 90 | Fat 7.4 g | Carbohydrates 10.1 g | Sugar 4.1 g | Protein 1 g | Cholesterol 0 mg

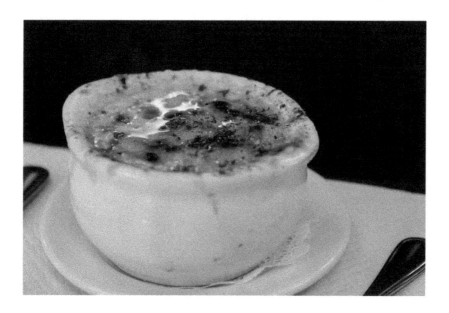

Avocado Broccoli Soup

Preparation Time: 25 minutes | Cooking Time: 15-60 minutes |
Servings: 4

Ingredients:

• 2 cups broccoli florets, chopped

• 5 cups vegetable broth

• 2 avocados, chopped

• Pepper

• Salt

Directions:

• Cook broccoli in boiling water for 5 minutes. Drain well.

• Add broccoli, vegetable broth, avocados, pepper, and salt to
the blender and blend until smooth.

• Stir well and serve warm.

Nutrition:

Calories 269 | Fat 21.5 g | Carbohydrates 12.8 g | Sugar 2.1 g |
Protein 9.2 g | Cholesterol 0 mg

Green Spinach Kale Soup

Preparation Time: 15 minutes | Cooking Time: 15-60 minutes | Servings: 6

Ingredients:

- 2 avocados

- 8 oz spinach

- 8 oz kale

- 1 fresh lime juice

- 1 cup of water

- 3 1/3 cup coconut milk

- 3 oz olive oil

- 1/4 tsp pepper

- 1 tsp salt

Directions:

- Heat olive oil in a saucepan over medium heat.

- Add kale and spinach to the saucepan and sauté for 2-3 minutes. Remove saucepan from

heat. Add coconut milk, spices, avocado, and water. Stir well.

- Puree the soup using an immersion blender until smooth and creamy. Add fresh lime juice

and stir well.

- Serve and enjoy.

Nutrition:

Calories 233 | Fat 20 g | Carbohydrates 12 g | Sugar 0.5 g | Protein 4.2 g | Cholesterol 0 mg

Cauliflower Asparagus Soup

Preparation Time: 30 minutes | Cooking Time: 15-60 minutes | Servings: 4

Ingredients:

- 20 asparagus spears, chopped

- 4 cups vegetable stock

- ½ cauliflower head, chopped

- 2 garlic cloves, chopped

- 1 tbsp coconut oil

- Pepper

- Salt

Directions:

- Heat coconut oil in a large saucepan over medium heat.

- Add garlic and sauté until softened.

- Add cauliflower, vegetable stock, pepper, and salt. Stir well and bring to boil.

• Reduce heat to low and simmer for 20 minutes.

• Add chopped asparagus and cook until softened.

• Puree the soup using an immersion blender until smooth and creamy.

• Stir well and serve warm.

Nutrition:

Calories 74 | Fat 5.6 g | Carbohydrates 8.9 g | Sugar 5.1 g | Protein 3.4 g | Cholesterol 2 mg

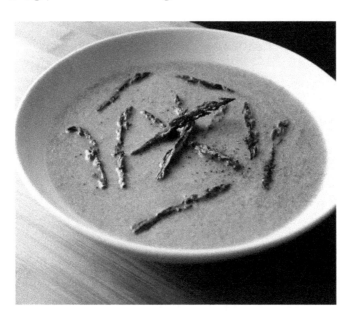

African Pineapple Peanut Stew

Preparation Time: 30 mins. | Cooking Time: 15-60 minutes | Servings: 4

Ingredients:

- 4 cups sliced kale

- 1 cup chopped onion

- ½ cup peanut butter

- 1 tbsp. hot pepper sauce or 1 tbsp. Tabasco sauce

- 2 minced garlic cloves

- ½ cup chopped cilantro

- 2 cups pineapple, undrained, canned & crushed

- 1 tbsp. vegetable oil

Directions:

- In a saucepan (preferably covered), sauté the garlic and onions in the oil until the onions are lightly browned, approximately 10 minutes, stirring often.

• Wash the kale. Get rid of the stems. Mound the leaves on a cutting surface & slice crosswise into slices (preferably 1‖ thick).

• Now put the pineapple and juice to the onions & bring to a simmer. Stir the kale in, cover, and simmer until just tender, stirring frequently for approximately 5 minutes.

• Mix in the hot pepper sauce, peanut butter & simmer for another 5 minutes.

• Add salt according to your taste.

Nutrition:

382 Calories | 20.3 g Total Fat | 0 mg Cholesterol | 27.6 g Total Carbohydrate | 5 g Dietary Fiber | 11.4 g Protein

Fuss-Free Cabbage and Tomatoes Stew

Preparation Time: 15-30 minutes | Cooking Time: 3 hours and 10 minutes | Servings: 6

Ingredients:

- 1 medium-sized cabbage head, chopped

- 1 medium-sized white onion, peeled and sliced

- 28-ounce of stewed tomatoes

- 3/4 teaspoon of salt

- 1/4 teaspoon of ground black pepper

- 10-ounce of tomato soup

Directions:

- Using a 6 quarts slow cooker, place all the ingredients, and stir properly.

- Cover it with the lid, plug in the slow cooker and let it cook at the high heat setting for 3 hours or until the vegetables get soft.

- Serve right away.

Nutrition:

Calories:103 Cal | Carbohydrates:17g | Protein:4g | Fats:2g |
Fiber:4g.

Awesome Spinach Artichoke Soup

Preparation Time: 15-30 minutes | Cooking Time: 4 hours and 45 minutes | Servings: 6

Ingredients:

• 15 ounce of cooked white beans

 • 2 cups of frozen artichoke hearts, thawed

• 2 cups of spinach leaves

• 1 small red onion, peeled and chopped

• 1 teaspoon of minced garlic

• 1 teaspoon of salt

• 1/2 teaspoon of ground black pepper

• 2 teaspoons of dried basil

• 1 teaspoon of dried oregano

• 1/2 teaspoon of whole-grain mustard paste

• 2 1/2 tablespoons of nutritional yeast

• 1 1/2 teaspoons of white miso

- 4 tablespoons of lemon juice

- 16 fluid ounce of almond milk, unsweetened

- 3 cups of vegetable broth

- 1 cups of water

Directions:

• Grease a 6-quarts slow cooker with a non-stick cooking spray, add the artichokes, spinach, onion, garlic, salt, black pepper, basil, and oregano.

• Pour in the vegetable broth and water, stir properly and cover it with the lid.

• Then plug in the slow cooker and let it cook at the high heat setting for 4 hours or until the vegetables get soft.

• While waiting for that, place the white beans in a food processor, add the yeast, miso, mustard, lemon juice, and almond milk.

• Mash until it gets smooth, and set it aside.

• When the vegetables are cooked thoroughly, add the prepared bean mixture and continue cooking for 30 minutes at the high heat setting or until the soup gets slightly thick.

• Garnish it with cheese and serve.

Nutrition:

Calories:200 Cal | Carbohydrates:13g | Protein:4g | Fats:12g | Fiber:2g.

Brazilian Black Bean Stew

Preparation Time: 15 minutes | Cooking Time: 30 minutes | Servings: 2

Ingredients:

- ½ tablespoon olive oil

- 1 medium onion, chopped

- 1 teaspoon garlic powder

- ½ cup sweet potatoes, peeled and diced

- ½ large red bell pepper, diced

- 1 cup diced tomatoes with juice

- ½ cup of corn

- ½ cup broccoli

- 1 small hot green chili pepper, diced

- 1 1/2 cups water

- ½ cup black beans

- 1 mango - peeled, seeded, and diced

- ¼ cup chopped fresh cilantro

- ¼ teaspoon salt

Directions:

• Select the Sauté setting on the Pressure pot. Add olive oil and onions to the Pressure pot. Stir in garlic powder, and cook until tender, then mix in the sweet potatoes, bell pepper, tomatoes with juice, chili pepper, corn, broccoli, and water.

• Stir the beans into the Pressure pot. Select Pressure Cook or Manual, and adjust the pressure to High and the time to 12 minutes. After cooking, let the pressure release naturally for 10 minutes, then quickly release any remaining pressure.

• Open the lid and mix in the mango and cilantro, and season with salt.

Nutrition:

Calories 434 | Total Fat 5. 8g | Saturated Fat 1g | Cholesterol 0mg | Sodium 325mg | Total Carbohydrate 86. 6g | Dietary Fiber 16. 1g | Total Sugars 32. 4g | Protein 16. 3g

Split Pea and Carrot Stew

Preparation Time: 10 minutes | Cooking Time: 20 minutes | Servings: 2

Ingredients:

- 1 tablespoon avocado oil

- 1 small onion, diced

- ½ carrot, diced into small cubes

- ½ leek stick, diced into cubes

- 4–5 cloves garlic, diced finely

- 1 bay leaf

- 1 teaspoon paprika powder

- 1 1/2 teaspoons cumin powder

- ½ teaspoon salt

- ¼ teaspoon cinnamon powder

- ¼ teaspoon chili powder or cayenne pepper

- 2 cups green split peas (rinsed well

- ½ cup chopped tinned tomatoes

- Juice of ½ lemon

- 2 cups vegetable stock

Directions:

• Press the Sauté key to the Pressure pot. Add the avocado oil, onions, carrots, and leeks and cook for 4 minutes, stirring a few times.

• Add the rest of the ingredients and stir. Cancel the Sauté function by pressing the Keep Warm/Cancel button.

• Place and lock the lid, make sure the steam releasing handle is pointing to Sealing. Press Manual and adjust to 10 minutes.

• Once the timer goes off, allow the pressure to release for 4-5 minutes and then use the Quickrelease method before opening the lid.

• Serve.

Nutrition:

Calories 337 | Total Fat 20. 5g | Saturated Fat 4. 2g | Cholesterol 0mg | Sodium 661mg | Total Carbohydrate 32. 6g | Dietary Fiber 16. 3g | Total Sugars 7. 9g | Protein 10g

Beans, Tomato & Corn Quesadillas

Preparation Time: 15-30 minutes | Cooking Time: 35 minutes | Servings: 4

Ingredients:

- 1 tsp olive oil

- 1 small onion, chopped

- ½ medium red bell pepper, deseeded and chopped

- 1 (7 oz) can chopped tomatoes

- 1 (7 oz) can black beans, drained and rinsed

- 1 (7 oz) can sweet corn kernels, drained

- 4 whole-wheat tortillas

- 1 cup grated plant-based cheddar cheese

Directions:

• Heat the olive oil in a medium skillet and sauté the onion and bell pepper until softened, 3 minutes.

• Mix in the tomatoes, black beans, sweet corn, and cook until the tomatoes soften, 10 minutes. Season with salt and black pepper.

• Heat another medium skillet over medium heat and lay in one tortilla. Spread a quarter of the tomato mixture on top, scatter a quarter of the plant cheese on the sauce, and cover with another tortilla. Cook until the cheese melts. Flip and cook further for 2 minutes.

• Transfer to a plate and make one more piece using the remaining ingredients.

• Cut each tortilla set into quarters and serve immediately.

Nutrition:

Calories 197 | Fats 6. 4g | Carbs 30. 2g | Protein 6. 6g

Spinach and Mashed Tofu Salad

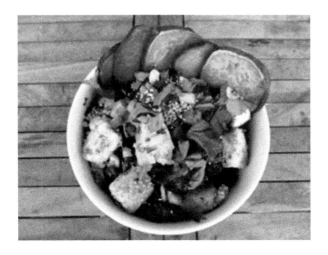

Preparation Time: 20 minutes | Cooking Time: 3-30 minutes | Servings: 4

Ingredients:

- 2 8-oz. blocks firm tofu, drained

- 4 cups baby spinach leaves

- 4 tbsp. cashew butter

- 1½ tbsp. soy sauce

- inch piece ginger, finely chopped

- 1 tsp. red miso paste

- 2 tbsp. sesame seeds

- 1 tsp. organic orange zest

- 1 tsp. nori flakes

- 2 tbsp. water

Directions:

- Use paper towels to absorb any excess water left in the tofu before crumbling both blocks into small pieces.

- In a large bowl, combine the mashed tofu with the spinach leaves.

- Mix the remaining ingredients in another small bowl and, if desired, add the optional water for a smoother dressing.

- Pour this dressing over the mashed tofu and spinach leaves.

- Transfer the bowl to the fridge and allow the salad to chill for up to one hour. Doing so will guarantee a better flavor. Or, the salad can be served right away. Enjoy!

Nutrition:

Calories 166 | Carbohydrates 5. 5 g | Fats 10. 7 g | Protein 11. 3 g

Cucumber Edamame Salad

Preparation Time: 5 minutes | Cooking Time: 8 minutes | Servings: 2

Ingredients:

- 3 tbsp. avocado oil

- 1 cup cucumber, sliced into thin rounds

- ½ cup fresh sugar snap peas, sliced or whole

- ½ cup fresh edamame

- ¼ cup radish, sliced

- 1 large Hass avocado, peeled, pitted, sliced

- 1 nori sheet, crumbled

- 2 tsp. roasted sesame seeds

- 1 tsp. salt

Directions:

- Bring a medium-sized pot filled halfway with water to a boil over medium-high heat.

• Add the sugar snaps and cook them for about 2 minutes.

• Take the pot off the heat, drain the excess water, transfer the sugar snaps to a medium-sized bowl, and set aside for now.

• Fill the pot with water again, add the teaspoon of salt and bring to a boil over medium-high heat.

• Add the edamame to the pot and let them cook for about 6 minutes.

• Take the pot off the heat, drain the excess water, transfer the soybeans to the bowl with sugar snaps, and let them cool down for about 5 minutes.

• Combine all ingredients, except the nori crumbs and roasted sesame seeds, in a medium sized bowl.

• Carefully stir, using a spoon, until all ingredients are evenly coated in oil.

• Top the salad with the nori crumbs and roasted sesame seeds.

• Transfer the bowl to the fridge and allow the salad to cool for at least 30 minutes. Serve chilled and enjoy!

Nutrition:

Calories 409 | Carbohydrates 7. 1 g | Fats 38. 25 g | Protein 7. 6 g

Artichoke White Bean Sandwich Spread

Preparation Time: 10 minutes | Cooking Time: 3-30 minutes | Servings: 2

Ingredients:

- ½ cup raw cashews, chopped

- Water

- 1 clove garlic, cut into half

- 1 tablespoon lemon zest

- 1 teaspoon fresh rosemary, chopped

- ¼ teaspoon salt

- ¼ teaspoon pepper

- 6 tablespoons almond, soy, or coconut milk

- 1 15. 5-ounce can cannellini beans, rinsed and drained well

- 3 to 4 canned artichoke hearts, chopped

- ¼ cup hulled sunflower seeds

- Green onions, chopped, for garnish

Directions:

• Soak the raw cashews for 15 minutes in enough water to cover them. Drain and dab with a paper towel to make them as dry as possible.

• Transfer the cashews to a blender and add the garlic, lemon zest, rosemary, salt, and pepper. Pulse to break everything up and then add the milk, one tablespoon at a time, until the mixture is smooth and creamy.

• Mash the beans in a bowl with a fork. Add the artichoke hearts and sunflower seeds. Toss to mix.

• Pour the cashew mixture on top and season with more salt and pepper if desired. Mix the ingredients well and spread on whole-wheat bread, crackers, or a wrap.

Nutrition:

Calories 110 | Carbohydrates 14 g | Fats 4 g | Protein 6 g

Buffalo Chickpea Wraps

Preparation Time: 20 minutes | Cooking Time: 5 minutes | Servings: 4

Ingredients:

- ¼ cup plus 2 tablespoons hummus

- 2 tablespoons lemon juice

- 1½ tablespoons maple syrup

- 1 to 2 tablespoons hot water

- 1 head Romaine lettuce, chopped

- 1 15-ounce can chickpeas, drained, rinsed, and patted dry

- 4 tablespoons hot sauce, divided

- 1 tablespoon olive or coconut oil

- ¼ teaspoon garlic powder

- 1 pinch sea salt

- 4 wheat tortillas

- ¼ cup cherry tomatoes, diced

- ¼ cup red onion, diced

- ¼ of a ripe avocado, thinly sliced

Directions:

• Mix the hummus with lemon juice and maple syrup in a large bowl. Use a whisk and add the hot water, a little at a time until it is thick but spreadable.

• Add the Romaine lettuce and toss to coat. Set aside.

• Pour the prepared chickpeas into another bowl. Add three tablespoons of the hot sauce, olive oil, garlic powder, and salt; toss to coat.

• Heat a metal skillet (cast iron works the best) over medium heat and add the chickpea mixture. Sauté for three to five minutes and mash gently with a spoon.

• Once the chickpea mixture is slightly dried out, remove it from the heat and add the rest of the hot sauce. Stir it in well and set aside.

• Lay the tortillas on a clean, flat surface and spread a quarter cup of the buffalo chickpeas on top. Top with tomatoes, onion, and avocado (optional) and wrap.

Nutrition:

Calories 254 | Carbohydrates 39. 4 g | Fats 6. 7 g | Protein 9. 1 g

Coconut Veggie Wraps

Preparation Time: 5 minutes | Cooking Time: 3-30 minutes | Servings: 5

Ingredients:

- 1½ cups shredded carrots

- 1 red bell pepper, seeded, thinly sliced

- 2½ cups kale

- 1 ripe avocado, thinly sliced

- 1 cup fresh cilantro, chopped

- 5 coconut wraps

- 2/3 cups hummus

- 6½ cups green curry paste

Directions:

- Slice, chop, and shred all the vegetables.

- Lay a coconut wrap on a clean flat surface and spread two tablespoons of the hummus and one tablespoon of the green curry paste on top of the end closest to you.

• Place some carrots, bell pepper, kale, and cilantro on the wrap and start rolling it up, starting from the edge closest to you. Roll tightly and fold in the ends.

• Place the wrap, seam down, on a plate to serve.

Nutrition:

Calories 236 | Carbohydrates 23. 6 g | Fats 14. 3 g | Protein 5. 5 g

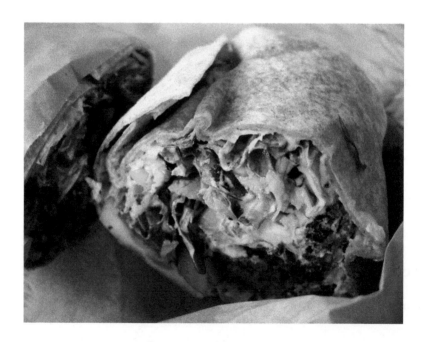

Cucumber Avocado Sandwich

Preparation Time: 15 minutes | Cooking Time: 3-30 minutes | Servings: 2

Ingredients:

• ½ of a large cucumber, peeled, sliced

• ¼ teaspoon salt

• 4 slices whole-wheat bread

• 4 ounces goat cheese with or without herbs, at room temperature

• 2 Romaine lettuce leaves

• 1 large avocado, peeled, pitted, sliced

• 2 pinches lemon pepper

• 1 squeeze of lemon juice

• ½ cup alfalfa sprouts

Directions:

• Peel and slice the cucumber thinly. Lay the slices on a plate and sprinkle them with a quarter to a half teaspoon of salt. Let this sit for 10 minutes or until water appears on the plate.

• Place the cucumber slices in a colander and rinse with cold water. Let these drain, then place them on a dry plate and pat dry with a paper towel.

• Spread all slices with goat cheese and place lettuce leaves on the two bottom pieces of bread.

• Layer the cucumber slices and avocado atop the bread.

• Sprinkle one pinch of lemon pepper over each sandwich and drizzle a little lemon juice over the top.

• Top with the alfalfa sprouts and place another piece of bread, goat cheese down, on top.

Nutrition:

Calories 246 | Carbohydrates 20 g | Fats 12 g | Protein 9 g

Fresh Puttanesca With Quinoa

Preparation Time: 15-30 minutes | Cooking Time: 30 minutes | Servings: 4

Ingredients:

- 1 cup brown quinoa

- 2 cups of water

- 1/8 tsp salt

- 4 cups plum tomatoes, chopped

- 4 pitted green olives, sliced

- 4 pitted Kalamata olives, sliced

- 1 ½ tbsp capers, rinsed and drained

- 2 garlic cloves, minced

- 1 tbsp olive oil

- 1 tbsp chopped fresh parsley

- ¼ cup chopped fresh basil

- 1/8 tsp red chili flakes

Directions:

• Add the quinoa, water, and salt to a medium pot and cook covered over medium heat until tender and water is absorbed for about 10 to 15 minutes.

• Meanwhile, in a medium bowl, mix the tomatoes, green olives, Kalamata olives, capers, garlic, olive oil, parsley, basil, and red chili flakes. Allow sitting for 5 minutes.

• Serve the puttanesca with the quinoa.

Nutrition:

Calories 427 kcal | Fats 7. 1g | Carbs 88. 2g | Protein 7. 2g

Quinoa Cherry Tortilla Wraps

Preparation Time: 15-30 minutes | Cooking Time: 25 minutes | Servings: 4

Ingredients:

- ½ cup brown quinoa

- Salt and black pepper to taste

- 2 tsp olive oil

- 1 ½ cups shredded carrots

- 1 ¼ cups fresh cherries, pitted and halved

- 4 scallions, chopped

- 2 tbsp plain vinegar

- 2 tbsp low-sodium soy sauce

- 1 tbsp pure maple syrup

- 4 (8-inch) tortilla wraps

Directions:

• Cook the quinoa in 1 cup of slightly salted water in a medium pot over medium heat until tender and the water absorbs, 10 minutes. Fluff and set aside to warm.

• Heat the olive oil in a medium skillet and sauté the carrots, cherries, and scallions. While cooking, in a small bowl, mix the vinegar, soy sauce, and maple syrup. Stir the mixture into the vegetable mixture. Simmer for 5 minutes and turn the heat off.

• Spread the tortillas on a flat surface, spoon the mixture at the center, fold the sides and ends to wrap in the filling.

• Serve warm.

Nutrition:

Calories 282 kcal | Fats 6. 5g | Carbs 48g | Protein 8. 3g

Quinoa with Mixed Herbs

Preparation Time: 15-30 minutes | Cooking Time: 20 minutes | Servings: 4

Ingredients:

• 1 cup quinoa, well-rinsed

• 2 cups vegetable broth

• Salt to taste

• 2 garlic cloves, minced, divided

• ¼ cup chopped chives

• 2 tbsp finely chopped parsley

• 2 tbsp finely chopped basil

• 2 tbsp finely chopped mint

• 2 tbsp finely chopped soft sundried tomatoes

• 1 tbsp olive oil (optional)

• ½ tsp lemon zest

• 1 tbsp fresh lemon juice

• 2 tbsp minced walnuts

• Salt and black pepper to taste

Directions:

• In a medium pot, combine the quinoa, vegetable broth, ¼ tsp of salt, and half of the garlic in a medium saucepan. Boil until the quinoa is tender and the liquid absorbs, 10-15 minutes. • Open the lid, fluff with a fork, and stir in the chives, parsley, basil, mint, tomatoes, olive oil, zest, lemon juice, and walnuts. Warm for 5 minutes.

• Dish the food and serve warm.

Nutrition:

Calories 393 kcal | Fats 17. 1g | Carbs 31. 9g | Protein 27. 8g

Chickpea Avocado Pizza

Preparation Time: 15-30 minutes | Cooking Time: 40 minutes | Servings: 4

Ingredients:

For the pizza crust:

- 3 ½ cups whole-wheat flour

- 1 tsp yeast

- 1 tsp salt

- 1 pinch sugar

- 3 tbsp olive oil

- 1 cup of warm water

For the topping:

- 1 cup red pizza sauce

- 1 cup baby spinach

- Salt and black pepper to taste

- 1 (15 oz) can chickpeas, drained and rinsed

- 1 medium avocado, pitted, peeled, and chopped

- ¼ cup grated plant-based Parmesan cheese

Directions:

- Preheat the oven the 350 F and lightly grease a pizza pan with cooking spray.

- In a medium bowl, mix the flour, nutritional yeast, salt, sugar, olive oil, and warm water until smooth dough forms. Allow rising for an hour or until the dough doubles in size.

- Spread the dough on the pizza pan and apply the pizza sauce on top.

- Top with the spinach, chickpeas, avocado, and plant Parmesan cheese.

- Bake the pizza for 20 minutes or until the cheese melts.

- Remove from the oven, cool for 5 minutes, slice, and serve.

Nutrition:

Calories 678 kcal | Fats 22. 7g | Carbs 104. 1g | Protein 23. 5g

White Bean Stuffed Squash

Preparation Time: 15-30 minutes | Cooking Time: 60 minutes | Servings: 4

Ingredients:

- 2 pounds large acorn squash

- 2 tbsp olive oil

- 3 garlic cloves, minced

- 1 (15 oz) can white beans, drained and rinsed

- 1 cup chopped spinach leaves

- ½ cup vegetable stock

- Salt and black pepper to taste

- ½ tsp cumin powder

- ½ tsp chili powder

Directions:

- Preheat the oven to 350 F.

- Cut the squash into half and scoop out the seeds.

• Season with salt and pepper and place face down on a sheet pan. Bake for 45 minutes.

• While the squash cooks, heat the olive oil in a medium pot over medium heat.

• Sauté the garlic until fragrant, 30 seconds, and mix in the beans. Cook for 1 minute.

• Stir in the spinach, allow wilting for 2 minutes, and season with salt, black pepper, cumin powder, and chili powder. Cook for 2 minutes and turn the heat off.

• When the squash is fork-tender, remove it from the oven and fill the holes with the bean and spinach mixture.

• Serve warm.

Nutrition:

Calories 365 kcal | Fats 34. 6g | Carbs 16. 7g | Protein 2. 3g

Grilled Zucchini and Spinach Pizza

Preparation Time: 15-30 minutes | Cooking Time: 30 minutes | Servings: 4

Ingredients:

- For the pizza crust:

- 3 ½ cups whole-wheat flour

- 1 tsp yeast

- 1 tsp salt

- 1 pinch sugar

- 3 tbsp olive oil

- 1 cup of warm water

- For the topping:

- 1 cup marinara sauce

- 2 large zucchinis, sliced

- ½ cup chopped spinach

- ¼ cup pitted and sliced black olives

- ½ cup grated plant Parmesan cheese

Directions:

- Preheat the oven the 350 F and lightly grease a pizza pan with cooking spray.

- In a medium bowl, mix the flour, nutritional yeast, salt, sugar, olive oil, and warm water until

smooth dough forms. Allow rising for an hour or until the dough doubles in size. Spread the dough on the pizza pan and apply the pizza sauce on top.

- Meanwhile, heat a grill pan over medium heat, season the zucchinis with salt, black pepper, and cook in the pan until slightly charred on both sides.

- Set the cucumbers on the pizza crust and top with the spinach, olives, and plant Parmesan cheese. Bake the pizza for 20 minutes or until the cheese melts. Remove from the oven, cool for 5 minutes, slice, and serve.

Nutrition:

Calories 519 kcal | Fats 13. 4g | Carbs 87. 5g | Protein 19. 6g

Honey-Almond Popcorn

Preparation Time: 5 minutes | Cooking Time: 10 minutes | Servings: 4

Ingredients:

- 1/2 cup popcorn kernels

- 2 tablespoons honey

- 1/2 teaspoon sea salt

- 2 tablespoons coconut sugar

- 1 cup roasted almonds

- 1/4 cup walnut oil

Directions:

• Take a pot, place it over medium-low heat, add oil and when it melts, add four kernels and wait until they sizzle.

• Then add the remaining kernel, toss until coated, sprinkle with sugar, drizzle with honey, shut the pot with the lid, and shake the kernels until popped completely, adding almonds halfway.

• Once all the kernels have popped, season them with salt and serve straight away.

Nutrition:

Calories: 120 Cal | Fat: 4.5 g | Carbs: 19 g | Protein: 1 g | Fiber: 1 g

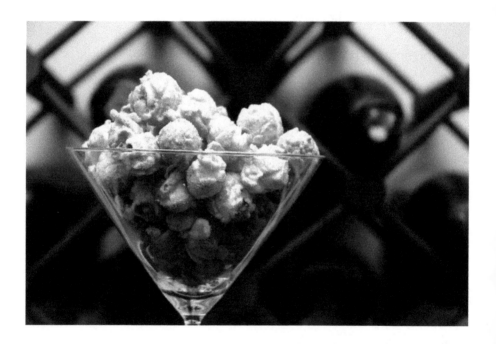

Turmeric Snack Bites

Preparation Time: 35 minutes | Cooking Time: 0 minute | Servings: 10

Ingredients:

- 1 cup Medjool dates, pitted, chopped

- 1/2 cup walnuts

- 1 teaspoon ground turmeric

- 1 tablespoon cocoa powder, unsweetened

- 1/2 teaspoon ground cinnamon

- 1/2 cup shredded coconut, unsweetened

Directions:

- Place all the ingredients in a food processor and pulse for 2 minutes until a smooth mixture comes together.

- Tip the mixture in a bowl and then shape it into ten small balls, 1 tablespoon of the mixture per ball and then refrigerate for 30 minutes.

- Serve straight away.

Nutrition:

Calories: 109 Cal | Fat: 2 g | Carbs: 13 g | Protein: 1 g | Fiber: 0 g

Watermelon Pizza

Preparation Time: 10 minutes | Cooking Time: 0 minute | Servings: 10

Ingredients:

- 1/2 cup strawberries, halved

- 1/2 cup blueberries

- 1 watermelon

- 1/2 cup raspberries

- 1 cup of coconut yogurt

- 1/2 cup pomegranate seeds

- 1/2 cup cherries

- Maple syrup as needed

Directions:

• Cut watermelon into 3-inch-thick slices, then spread yogurt on one side, leaving some space in the edges, and then top evenly with fruits and drizzle with maple syrup.

• Cut the watermelon into wedges and then serve.

Nutrition:

• Calories: 150 Cal | Fat: 4 g | Carbs: 21 g | Protein: 10 g | Fiber: 2 g

Nooch Popcorn

Preparation Time: 10 minutes | Cooking Time: 10 minutes | Servings: 4

Ingredients:

- 1/3 cup nutritional yeast

- 1 teaspoon of sea salt

- 3 tablespoons coconut oil

- ½ cup popcorn kernels

Directions:

- Place yeast in a large bowl, stir in salt and set aside until required.

- Take a medium saucepan, place it over medium-high heat, add oil and when it melts, add four kernels and wait until they sizzle.

- Then add the remaining kernel, toss until coated, shut the pan with the lid, and shake the kernels until popped completely.

- When done, transfer popcorn to the yeast mixture, shut with lid, and shape well until coated.

• Serve straight away

Nutrition:

Calories: 160 Cal | Fat: 6 g | Carbs: 28 g | Protein: 3 g | Fiber: 4 g

Masala Popcorn

Preparation Time: 5 minutes | Cooking Time: 15 minutes | Servings: 4

Ingredients:

- 3 cups popped popcorn

- 2 hot chili peppers, sliced

- 1 teaspoon ground cumin

- 6 curry leaves

- 1 teaspoon ground coriander

- 1/3 teaspoon salt

- 1/8 teaspoon chaat masala

- 1/4 teaspoon turmeric powder

- ¼ teaspoon red pepper flakes

- 1/4 teaspoon garam masala

- 1/3 cup olive oil

Directions:

• Take a large pot, place it over medium heat, add half of the oil and when hot, add chili peppers and curry leaves and cook for 3 minutes until golden.

• When done, transfer curry leaves and pepper to a plate lined with paper towels and set aside until required.

• Add remaining oil into the pot, add remaining ingredients except for popcorns, stir until mixed and cook for 1 minute until fragrant.

• Then tip in popcorns, remove the pan from heat, stir well until coated, and then sprinkle with bay leaves and red chili.

• Toss until mixed and serve straight away.

Nutrition:

Calories: 150 Cal | Fat: 9 g | Carbs: 15 g | Protein: 2 g | Fiber: 4 g

Cauliflower Nuggets

Preparation Time: 35 minutes | Cooking Time: 0 minutes | Servings: 4

Ingredients:

- 3 tablespoon yeast flakes

- 60 ml of soy milk

- ½ cauliflower

- 2 tablespoons of oil

- ½ cup breadcrumbs

- 30 g flour

- Salt and pepper

Directions:

- Separate the cauliflower into florets and wash.

- Mix the flour, yeast flakes, milk, salt, and pepper.

- Roll the cauliflower in the mass and then roll in breadcrumbs.

- Place on a baking sheet and drizzle with oil.

- Bake for about 35 minutes at 200 degrees Celsius, until the cauliflower is cooked through.

Nutrition:

Calories: 279 | Fat: 15.4g| Carbs: 20.5g | Protein: 12.1g | Fiber: 3.2g

Cauliflower Potato Burgers

Preparation Time: 15 minutes | Cooking Time: 7 minutes | Servings: 2

Ingredients:

- 7 oz cauliflower rice
- 1/4 cup mashed potato
- 1 tablespoon almond flour
- 1 teaspoon salt
- 1 teaspoon white pepper
- 1 tablespoon coconut yogurt
- 1 tablespoon breadcrumbs
- 1/2 cup water, for cooking

Directions:

- In the mixing bowl combine cauliflower rice and mashed potato.
- Add almond flour, salt, white pepper, and coconut yogurt.

- Then wear gloves and make medium size burgers from the mixture.

- Sprinkle every burger with breadcrumbs and wrap it in the foil.

- Pour water into the Pressure pot bowl and insert the steamer rack.

- Place wrapped burgers on the steamer rack and close the lid.

- Cook the meal on High (Manual mode) for 7 minutes. Then allow natural pressure release for 10 minutes.

Nutrition:

Calories: 163 | Fat: 9 | Fiber: 4.8 | Carbs: 17 | Protein: 6.6

Sweet Potato Burgers

Preparation Time: 10 minutes | Cooking Time: 20 minutes | Servings: 2

Ingredients:

- 1 sweet potato

- 1/2 onion, diced

- 1 teaspoon chives

- 1/2 teaspoon salt

- 1 teaspoon cayenne pepper

- 3 tablespoon flax meal

- 1/2 cup kale

- 1 teaspoon olive oil

- 1/2 cup water, for cooking

Directions:

- Pour water into the Pressure pot and insert the steamer rack.

- Place sweet potato on the steamer rack and close the lid.

• Cook the vegetables on Manual mode (High pressure) for 15 minutes (quick pressure release).

• Meanwhile, place onion, chives, and kale in the blender. Blend until smooth.

• Transfer the blended mixture to the mixing bowl.

• When the sweet potato is cooked – cut it into halves and scoop all the flesh into the kale mixture. Mix it up carefully with the help of the fork.

• Add flax meal, salt, and cayenne pepper. Stir well.

• With the help of the fingertips make medium burgers.

• Clean the Pressure pot bowl and put olive oil inside.

• Preheat for 2-3 minutes on Sauté mode.

• Then add burgers and cook them for 2 minutes from each side on Sauté mode.

Nutrition:

Calories: 139 | Fat: 6.4 | Fiber: 6 | Carbs: 19.7 | Protein: 4.3

Potato Patties

Preparation Time: 10 minutes | Cooking Time: 15 minutes | Servings: 4

Ingredients:

- 3 russet potatoes, peeled

- 3 tablespoon aquafaba

- 1/2 teaspoon salt

- 1 teaspoon almond butter

- 1/2 teaspoon smoked paprika

- 1/4 teaspoon chili flakes

- 2 tablespoon wheat flour

Directions:

- With the help of the hand mixer, whisk aquafaba until you get soft peaks.

- Then grate potatoes and combine them with aquafaba in the mixing bowl.

• Add salt, smoked paprika, chili flakes, and wheat flour. Mix it up carefully.

• Preheat the Pressure pot on Sauté mode for 4 minutes. Add almond butter and melt it.

• Then with the help of the spoon make medium patties; press them a little with the help of hand palms and put in the hot almond butter.

• Cook the patties for 3 minutes then flip into another side. Cook the patties for 4 minutes more.

Nutrition:

Calories: 150 | Fat: 2.5 | Fiber: 4.4 | Carbs: 29 | Protein: 4

Lentil Burgers

Preparation Time: 20 minutes | Cooking Time: 26 minutes | Servings: 7

Ingredients:

• 1 cup lentils, soaked overnight

• 1 cup of water

• 1/2 carrot, peeled

• 1 teaspoon cayenne pepper

• 4 tablespoon wheat flour

• 1 teaspoon salt

• 1 teaspoon olive oil

• 1 tablespoon dried dill

Directions:

• Put lentils in the Pressure pot together with water, carrot, salt, and cayenne pepper.

• Close the lid and set Manual mode (High pressure).

- Cook the ingredients for 25 minutes and allow natural pressure release for 10 minutes.

- Transfer the cooked ingredients in the blender and blend until smooth.

- Add wheat flour and dried dill. Mix it up until smooth. If the mixture is liquid – add more flour.

- Make the burgers and place them together with the olive oil in the Pressure pot.

- Set Manual mode (High pressure) for 1 minute (quick pressure release).

- It is recommended to serve burgers warm.

Nutrition:

Calories 122 | Fat 1.1 | Fiber 8.7 | Carbs 20.7 | Protein 7.7

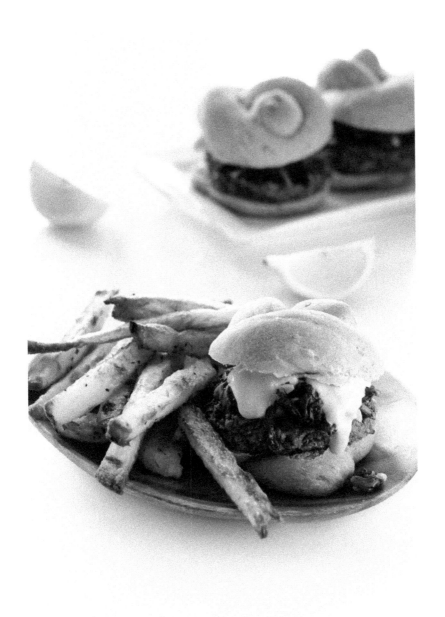

Lightning Source UK Ltd.
Milton Keynes UK
UKHW020801110621
385329UK00001B/166

9 781802 775235